SMOOTHIES TO PREVENT CANCER

The top 15 ingredients for smoothies that prevent cancer

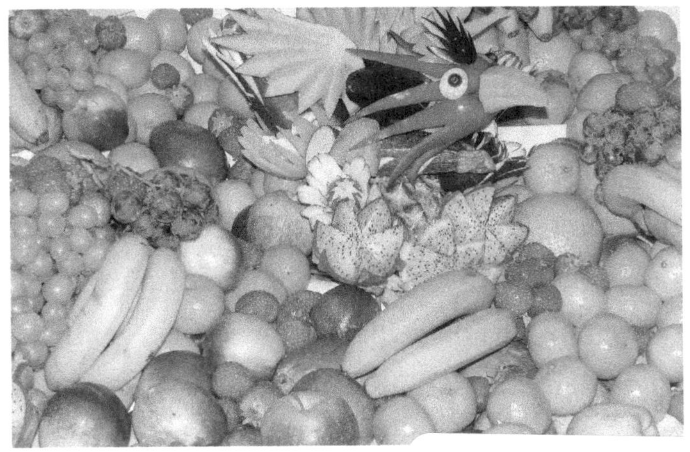

Carole R.Fortin

TABLE OF CONTENT

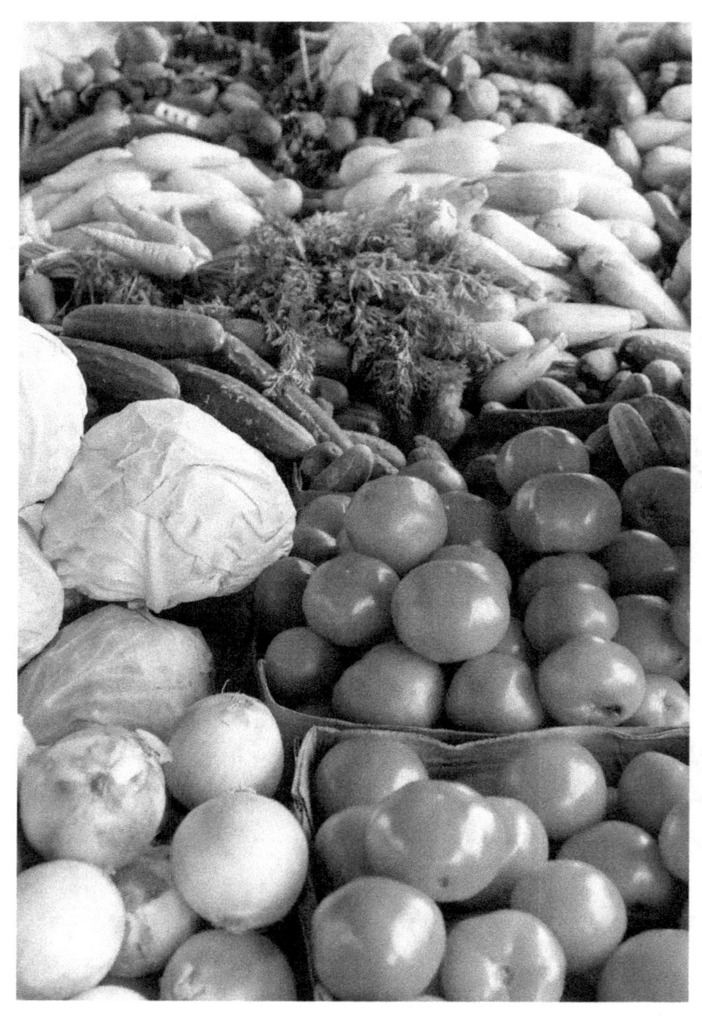

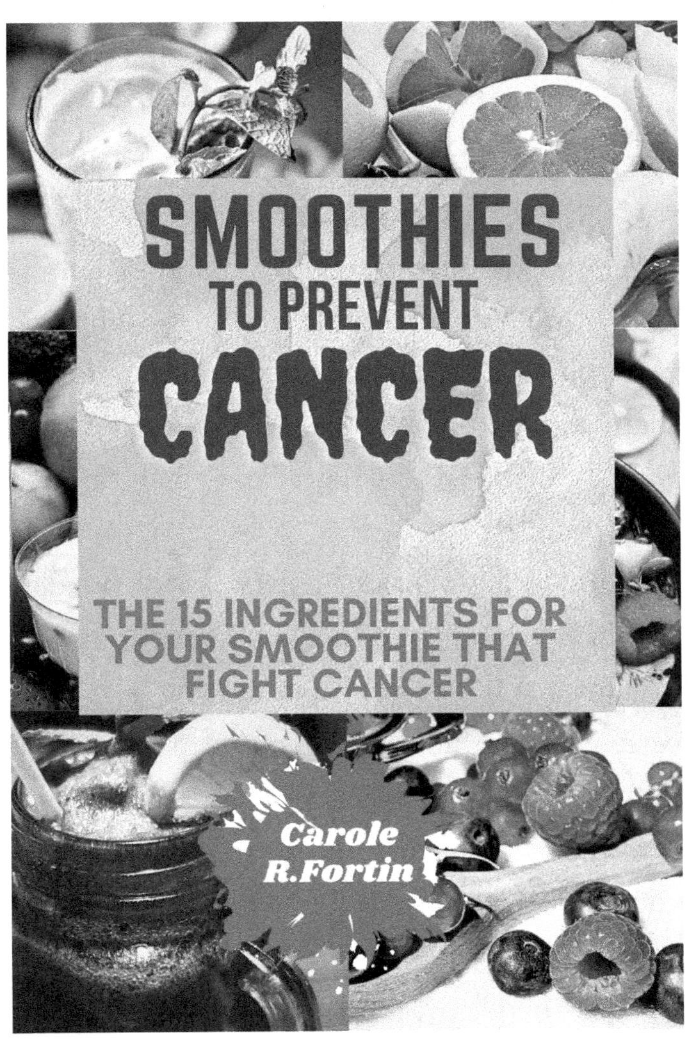

SMOOTHIES
TO PREVENT
CANCER
THE 15 INGREDIENTS FOR
YOUR SMOOTHIE THAT
FIGHT CANCER
Carole
R.Fortin

Introduction

Throughout the world, millions of people suffer from cancer. Even though there are many different treatment choices, prevention is always preferable to treatment. In recent years, researchers have identified several ingredients that can help prevent cancer. And what better way to consume these ingredients than through smoothies?

Smoothies have become increasingly popular as a healthy and convenient way to get a variety of nutrients in one glass. But did you know that certain smoothie ingredients can also help prevent cancer? By incorporating these ingredients into your daily smoothie routine, you can give your body the best chance at staying healthy.

In this book, we will explore the 15 best ingredients for smoothies that can help prevent cancer. Each ingredient has been carefully selected based on its proven anti-cancer properties and nutritional benefits. From leafy greens to berries, we'll cover a wide range of ingredients that will not only taste great but also help protect your body from cancer.

But this book is not just about recipes. We will also delve into the science behind each ingredient and explain how they work to prevent cancer. We'll provide tips on how to properly prepare and store your ingredients to ensure maximum nutritional value.

So whether you're a smoothie enthusiast or just looking for ways to improve your overall health, this book is for you. Let's get started on a journey to better health and cancer prevention, one smoothie at a time.

CHAPTER ONE

A brief overview of the importance of nutrition in cancer prevention and treatment

Nutrition plays a crucial role in both cancer prevention and treatment. A balanced and healthy diet that is rich in nutrients, fiber, and antioxidants can help reduce the risk of developing cancer and support the body's ability to fight the disease. On the other hand, a diet that is high in saturated fats, sugar, and processed foods may increase the risk of cancer.

For cancer patients, proper nutrition is essential to help manage the side effects of cancer treatments, such as nausea, vomiting, and loss of appetite. A well-balanced diet can also improve energy levels, support a healthy weight, and promote the healing and recovery process.

important dietary factors in cancer prevention and treatment

Eating a variety of fruits and vegetables to obtain a range of nutrients and antioxidants.

Choosing whole grains over refined carbohydrates to maintain a healthy blood sugar level.

Limiting the consumption of red and processed meats, which have been linked to an increased risk of some types of cancer.

eating fats that are good for you, such as those in nuts, seeds, and fatty fish.

Staying hydrated and avoiding sugary drinks.

Limiting alcohol consumption, which has been linked to an increased risk of certain cancers.

how smoothies can be a convenient and delicious way to incorporate cancer-fighting ingredients into one's diet

Smoothies can be an excellent way to incorporate cancer-fighting ingredients into one's diet. Smoothies are convenient because they can be made quickly and can be consumed on the go. They are also delicious and can be customized to one's preferences.

Many cancer-fighting ingredients can be added to smoothies, such as fruits, vegetables, and spices. For example, dark leafy greens such as kale and spinach are high in antioxidants and other nutrients that have been linked to a lower risk of cancer. Berries, such as blueberries and raspberries, contain antioxidants that can help protect cells from damage.

Turmeric is another ingredient that has been linked to cancer prevention. It contains curcumin, which has anti-inflammatory properties and may help prevent cancer cells from forming. Adding a teaspoon of turmeric to a smoothie can provide a delicious and convenient way to incorporate this ingredient into one's diet.

Other ingredients that can be added to smoothies for their cancer-fighting properties include ginger, garlic, and green tea. Ginger has anti-inflammatory properties that can help reduce inflammation in the body, while garlic contains compounds that have been shown to have anti-cancer properties. Green tea contains catechins, which are antioxidants that have been linked to a lower risk of cancer.

Juicing for health

Juicing is a popular method of consuming fruits and vegetables, either as a meal replacement or as a supplement to a healthy diet. Juicing involves extracting the juice from fresh fruits and vegetables using a juicer, leaving behind the fibrous pulp. The resulting juice is rich in vitamins, minerals, and other nutrients that are essential for maintaining good health.

Juicing has been promoted as a way to improve digestion, boost energy, and support overall health. Some proponents of juicing also claim that it can help prevent chronic diseases, such as cancer and heart disease. However, it is important to note that there is limited scientific evidence to support these claims.

One of the benefits of juicing is that it can help you consume a larger amount of fruits and vegetables than you would be able to eat in their whole form. This is because juicing removes the fiber, which can make it easier to consume a larger quantity of fruits and vegetables. However, it is important to note that fiber is an essential part of a healthy diet and should not be completely eliminated.

When juicing, it is important to use a variety of fruits and vegetables to ensure that you are getting a wide range of nutrients. Dark leafy greens, such as kale and spinach, are especially beneficial, as they are rich in vitamins and minerals that are essential for good health. Fruits such as berries and citrus fruits are also excellent choices for juicing, as they are high in antioxidants and other beneficial compounds.

While juicing can be a healthy addition to your diet, it is important to remember that it should not be used as a substitute for a balanced diet. Whole fruits and vegetables provide important fiber and other nutrients that are not found in juice. Additionally, consuming too much juice can lead to high sugar intake, which can be harmful to your health.

Best juicing vegetables

When it comes to juicing vegetables, there are several options that can provide a wide range of health benefits.

Kale - This leafy green is high in vitamins A, C, and K, as well as antioxidants and anti-inflammatory compounds.

Spinach - Another leafy green that is rich in vitamins and minerals, including iron, calcium, and magnesium.

Carrots - Carrots are high in beta-carotene, which can be converted to vitamin A in the body, and are also a good source of vitamin K and potassium.

Celery - Celery is low in calories and high in fiber, making it a good choice for weight loss. It is also a good source of vitamins A, C, and K, and minerals like potassium and folate.

Cucumbers - Cucumbers are a hydrating vegetable that can help support healthy skin and digestion. They are also low in calories and high in vitamin K and potassium.

Beets - Beets are a good source of fiber, folate, and potassium, and are also high in antioxidants that can help reduce inflammation in the body.

Ginger - While not a vegetable, ginger can be a beneficial addition to vegetable juice. It has anti-inflammatory properties and can help support digestion and immune function.

Flavor enhancer for juice

If you are looking for ways to enhance the flavor of your juice, there are several options that you can try:

Lemon or lime juice - Adding a small amount of fresh lemon or lime juice can help brighten the flavor of your juice and add a tangy, refreshing taste.

Fresh herbs - Herbs like mint, basil, and cilantro can add a fresh, aromatic flavor to your juice. Try adding a few leaves of your favorite herb to your juice and see how it tastes.

Ginger - Fresh ginger can add a spicy, warming flavor to your juice. Try adding a small piece of fresh ginger to your juice for a flavor boost.

Cinnamon - Ground cinnamon can add a sweet, warming flavor to your juice. Try adding a pinch of cinnamon to your juice for a cozy, comforting taste.

Apple or pear juice - If you find that your juice is too bitter or tart, adding a small amount of apple or pear juice can help balance the flavors and add a touch of sweetness.

Pineapple or mango - Adding a small amount of pineapple or mango to your juice can add a tropical, sweet flavor that compliments a variety of fruits and vegetables.

Watch Sugar Intake

Watching your sugar intake is important, even when consuming natural sugars from fruits and vegetables in juice form. While natural sugars are better for you than added sugars, they can still contribute to high blood sugar levels if consumed in excess.

To limit your sugar intake while still enjoying the benefits of fresh juice, here are some tips:

Use mostly vegetables in your juice - Vegetables tend to be lower in sugar than fruits, so using mostly vegetables in your juice can help keep the sugar content in check.

Limit high-sugar fruits - Fruits like bananas, grapes, and mangoes are high in sugar and can quickly increase the sugar content of your juice. Use these fruits sparingly, or choose lower-sugar options like berries, apples, and citrus fruits.

Add protein or fat - Adding protein or fat to your juice can help slow down the absorption of sugar into your bloodstream, which can help prevent spikes in blood sugar levels. Try adding a scoop of protein powder, a tablespoon of nut butter, or a handful of nuts or seeds to your juice.

Dilute your juice - Diluting your juice with water or ice can help lower the overall sugar content while still providing the benefits of fresh juice.

Monitor portion sizes - Drinking too much juice can quickly add up in terms of sugar and calories. Aim for 4-6 oz. serving size and enjoy your juice as a supplement to a healthy, balanced diet.

Advice about juicing to help with cancer treatment

If you are undergoing cancer treatment, juicing can be a helpful way to supplement your diet with extra nutrients and support your body's healing processes. However, it's important to work with your healthcare provider to ensure that juicing is safe and appropriate for your individual situation, as some types of cancer treatments can affect your digestion and nutrient absorption.

Here are some tips to consider when juicing in support of cancer treatment:

Consult with your healthcare provider - Talk to your doctor or dietitian before incorporating fresh juice into your diet. They can help you determine which fruits and vegetables are safe and appropriate for your individual needs, and help you monitor your nutrient intake.

Choose nutrient-dense fruits and vegetables - Choose fruits and vegetables that are high in vitamins, minerals, and antioxidants. This can include leafy greens, cruciferous vegetables, berries, citrus fruits, and more.

Avoid certain foods and supplements - Some foods and supplements can interfere with cancer treatment or cause negative side effects. Your healthcare provider can advise you on which foods and supplements to avoid during treatment.

Be mindful of food safety - When juicing at home, it's important to practice good food safety to avoid foodborne illness. Wash all fruits and vegetables thoroughly before juicing, and consume juice immediately after preparing to reduce the risk of bacterial growth.

Monitor your symptoms - If you experience any negative symptoms after consuming fresh juice, such as nausea, vomiting, or diarrhea, stop drinking juice and talk to your healthcare provider.

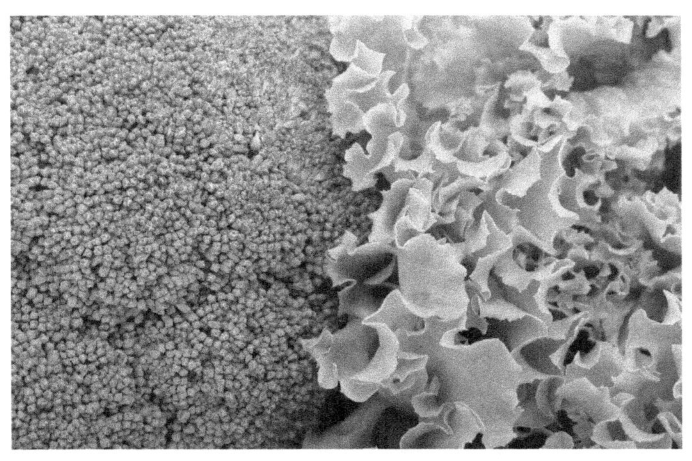

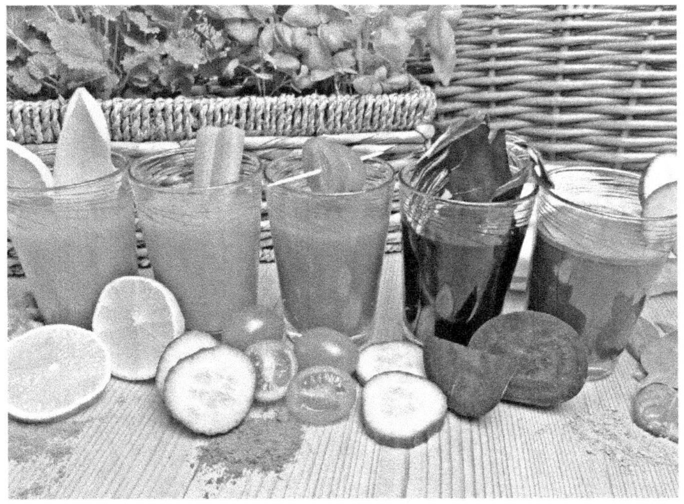

CHAPTER TWO

Berries

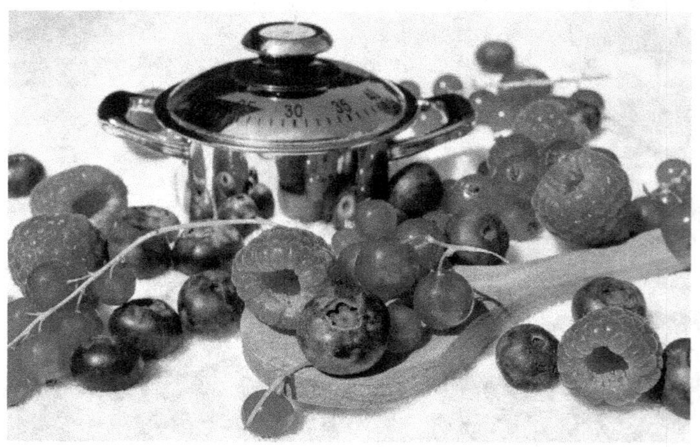

how berries contain powerful antioxidants and other compounds that have been shown to have anti-cancer effects

Berries are known for their delicious taste and vibrant colors, but they are also packed with powerful antioxidants and other compounds that have been shown to have anti-cancer effects. Antioxidants are molecules that can neutralize harmful molecules known as free radicals, which can cause damage to cells and DNA, leading to cancer and other diseases.

Berries are particularly high in a group of antioxidants known as anthocyanins, which give them their vibrant colors. These compounds have been shown to have a range of health benefits, including reducing inflammation, improving cardiovascular health, and protecting against cancer.

In addition to anthocyanins, berries also contain other important antioxidants such as vitamin C, vitamin E, and beta-carotene. These antioxidants work together to help protect cells from damage and reduce the risk of cancer.

Berries also contain other compounds that have been linked to anti-cancer effects. For example, ellagic acid, which is found in raspberries, strawberries, and blackberries, has been shown to have anti-cancer properties in animal studies. It works by blocking the production of enzymes that can cause cancer cells to grow and spread.

Another compound found in berries is resveratrol, which is found in grapes and berries such as blueberries and raspberries. Resveratrol has been shown to have anti-cancer effects in animal studies by reducing inflammation and inhibiting the growth and spread of cancer cells.

Berries contain powerful antioxidants such as anthocyanins, vitamin C, vitamin E, and beta-carotene, as well as other compounds such as ellagic acid and resveratrol, that have been shown to have anti-cancer effects. Incorporating berries into one's diet can be an easy and delicious way to obtain these health benefits and reduce the risk of cancer.

Specific berries to include in smoothies

There are several types of berries that are excellent choices to include in smoothies for their delicious taste and cancer-fighting properties. Here are some specific berries to consider adding to smoothies:

Blueberries: Blueberries are one of the most popular types of berries and for a good reason. They are high in antioxidants and other nutrients that can help protect against cancer. Additionally, a good source of fiber and vitamin C is blueberries.

Strawberries: Strawberries are another excellent choice for smoothies. They are high in vitamin C, folate, and potassium, and contain compounds that have been shown to have anti-cancer effects. Also low in calories and high in fiber are strawberries.

Raspberries: Raspberries are a good source of vitamin C, fiber, and antioxidants. They contain ellagic acid, a compound that has been shown to have anti-cancer effects. Raspberries are also low in calories and high in water content, making them a good choice for smoothies.

Blackberries: Blackberries are rich in antioxidants and other nutrients that can help protect against cancer. Additionally, they are an excellent source of fiber, vitamin C, and vitamin K.

Cranberries: Cranberries are another type of berry that can be added to smoothies. They are high in antioxidants and contain compounds that have been shown to help prevent urinary tract infections. Cranberries are also low in calories and high in fiber.

Leafy Greens

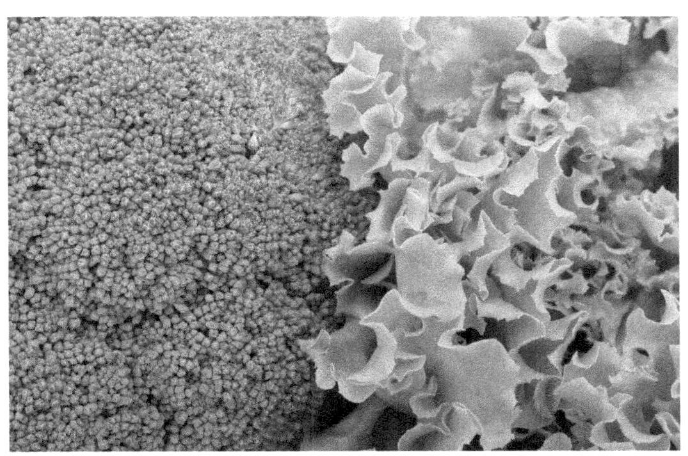

How leafy greens contain a variety of vitamins, minerals, and other nutrients that helps prevent cancer

Leafy greens are an excellent source of vitamins, minerals, and other nutrients that have been linked to a reduced risk of cancer. These vegetables are also low in calories and high in fiber, making them a great addition to any healthy diet.

Here are some of the key nutrients found in leafy greens that may help prevent cancer:

Antioxidants: Leafy greens are rich in antioxidants, including beta-carotene, vitamin C, and vitamin E. These antioxidants can help protect cells from damage caused by free radicals, which can lead to cancer.

Folate: Folate, also known as vitamin B9, is an essential nutrient found in leafy greens. A diet rich in fiber may lower the incidence of colorectal cancer, according to several research.

Fiber: Leafy greens are high in fiber, which can help promote healthy digestion and prevent constipation. Some studies have suggested that a diet high in fiber may reduce the risk of colorectal cancer.

Chlorophyll: Chlorophyll is the green pigment found in leafy greens. It has been shown to have anti-cancer properties in animal studies, although more research is needed to determine its effects in humans.

Carotenoids: Carotenoids are a group of antioxidants found in leafy greens. They include beta-carotene, lutein, and zeaxanthin. These compounds have been linked to a reduced risk of cancer, particularly lung and prostate cancer.

Vitamins and minerals: Leafy greens are also rich in vitamins and minerals such as vitamin K, vitamin A, and calcium, which are important for overall health and may also help prevent cancer.

Leafy greens are an excellent source of vitamins, minerals, and other nutrients that may help prevent cancer. They are low in calories, high in fiber, and can be easily incorporated into a variety of dishes, including smoothies, salads, and soups.

Specific greens to include in smoothies

There are several greens that you can include in your smoothies to make them healthy and delicious. Here are some options:

Spinach: Spinach is one of the most popular greens to include in smoothies. It is low in calories and high in nutrients, such as iron, calcium, and vitamins A and C.

Kale: Kale is another popular green to use in smoothies. It is also rich in nutrients, including iron, calcium, and vitamins A, C, and K.

Swiss chard: Swiss chard is a leafy green that is high in antioxidants and vitamins A and C. It has a slightly bitter taste, which can be balanced out with sweet fruits in a smoothie.

Arugula: Arugula is a peppery green that adds a nice flavor to smoothies. It is also rich in vitamins A, C, and K, as well as calcium and iron.

Collard greens: Collard greens are a good source of fiber, vitamin C, and calcium. They have a slightly bitter taste, which can be balanced out with sweet fruits.

Beet greens: The leaves of the beetroot plant are known as beet greens. They are high in iron, calcium, and vitamin K. They have a slightly bitter taste, which can be balanced out with sweet fruits.

Parsley: Parsley is a herb that is high in vitamin C, vitamin K, and antioxidants. Because of its strong taste, a little bit will go a long way.

These are just a few examples of the many greens you can use in smoothies. You can also experiment with other greens, such as dandelion greens, watercress, or even broccoli leaves. Just remember to wash them thoroughly before using them in your smoothies.

CHAPTER THREE

Cruciferous Vegetables

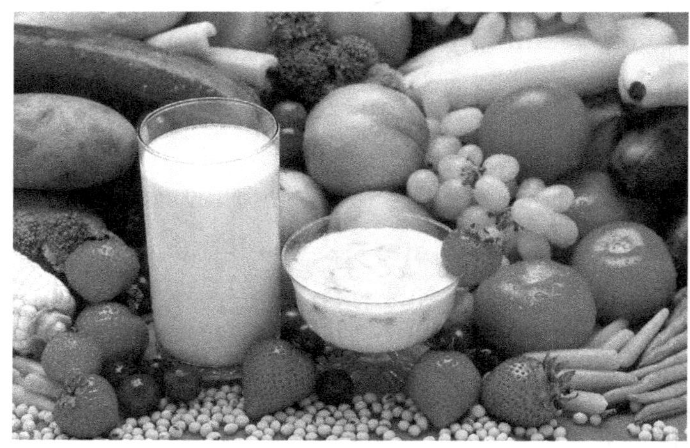

Explanation of how cruciferous vegetables contain compounds that have been shown to have anti-cancer effects

Cruciferous vegetables, such as broccoli, cauliflower, kale, and Brussels sprouts, contain compounds called glucosinolates. When these vegetables are chopped or chewed, the glucosinolates are broken down into several biologically active compounds, including isothiocyanates, indoles, and sulforaphane. Studies have shown that these compounds can have anti-cancer effects in several ways:

Inducing apoptosis: Apoptosis is a natural process by which damaged or abnormal cells are programmed to die. Some of the compounds in cruciferous vegetables have been shown to induce apoptosis in cancer cells.

Inhibiting cell cycle progression: Cancer cells divide rapidly, and the compounds in cruciferous vegetables can inhibit the progression of the cell cycle, which can slow down or prevent the growth of cancer cells.

Reducing inflammation: Chronic inflammation is associated with an increased risk of cancer. The compounds in cruciferous vegetables have been shown to reduce inflammation in the body.

Detoxifying carcinogens: Some of the compounds in cruciferous vegetables can help to detoxify carcinogens, which are substances that can cause cancer.

Inhibiting angiogenesis: Angiogenesis is the process by which tumors develop their own blood supply. Some of the compounds in cruciferous vegetables have been shown to inhibit angiogenesis, which can slow down or prevent the growth of tumors.

Overall, the anti-cancer effects of cruciferous vegetables are likely due to a combination of these mechanisms. Eating a diet rich in cruciferous vegetables has been associated with a reduced risk of several types of cancer, including lung, breast, colon, and prostate cancer.

Specific cruciferous vegetables to include in smoothies

While cruciferous vegetables are incredibly nutritious, they can be quite fibrous and may not blend well in smoothies. However, there are a few options that work well in smoothies and can add a nice flavor and nutrition boost. Here are some cruciferous vegetables you can include in your smoothies:

Broccoli sprouts: Sulforaphane, a substance with shown anti-cancer potential, is abundant in broccoli sprouts. They have a mild, slightly bitter taste and can be added to smoothies for an extra nutrition boost.

Baby kale: Baby kale is a milder form of kale that is less fibrous than mature kale. It has a slightly sweet taste and blends well in smoothies.

Baby bok choy: Baby bok choy is a Chinese cabbage that has a mild flavor and a high nutrient content. It is less fibrous than mature bok choy and can be blended into smoothies for a nutritional boost.

Watercress: Watercress is a peppery green that is rich in antioxidants and has anti-cancer properties. It has a strong flavor, so a little goes a long way in a smoothie.

Arugula: Arugula is another peppery green that adds a nice flavor to smoothies. It is high in vitamins A and C and has been shown to have anti-cancer properties.

When using cruciferous vegetables in smoothies, it's important to blend them well to ensure a smooth texture. You can also pair them with sweeter fruits or honey to balance out their slightly bitter taste.

Citrus Fruits

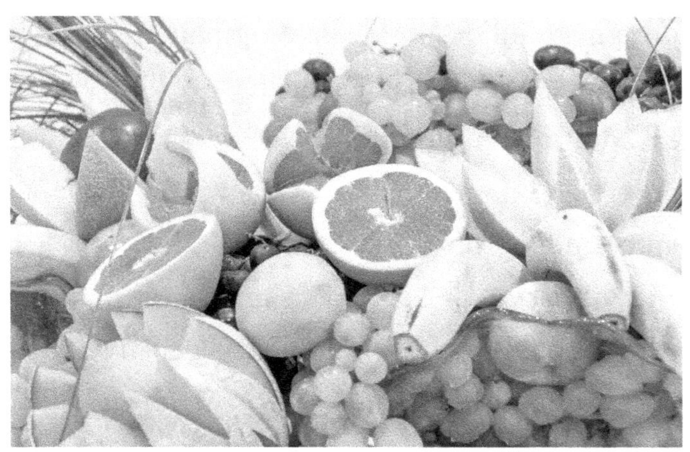

How citrus fruits contain compounds that helps to prevent cancer

Citrus fruits, such as oranges, lemons, limes, grapefruits, and tangerines, contain several compounds that have been shown to have anti-cancer properties.

One of the most studied compounds in citrus fruits is vitamin C, which is a powerful antioxidant that can protect cells from damage caused by free radicals. Free radicals are unstable molecules that can damage DNA, proteins, and other cellular components, which can increase the risk of cancer.

In addition to vitamin C, citrus fruits contain other compounds that have been shown to have anti-cancer properties. These include:

Flavonoids: Flavonoids are a group of compounds that are found in citrus fruits, as well as in other fruits and vegetables. They have antioxidant properties and can help to reduce inflammation, which can lower the risk of cancer.

Limonoids: Limonoids are compounds that are found in the peels and seeds of citrus fruits. They have been shown to have anti-cancer properties by inducing apoptosis (programmed cell death) in cancer cells.

Carotenoids: Citrus fruits also contain carotenoids, which are pigments that give fruits and vegetables their bright colors. Some carotenoids, such as beta-carotene and lycopene, have been shown to have anti-cancer properties.

Vitamin A: Citrus fruits are a good source of vitamin A, which is important for maintaining healthy skin and mucous membranes, as well as for promoting a healthy immune system.

Overall, the anti-cancer properties of citrus fruits are likely due to a combination of these compounds. Eating a diet rich in citrus fruits has been associated with a reduced risk of several types of cancer, including lung, breast, colon, and stomach cancer.

Specific citrus fruits to include in smoothies

Citrus fruits can add a refreshing and tangy flavor to smoothies, while also providing a variety of important nutrients. Here are some citrus fruits you can include in your smoothies:

Oranges: Oranges are a good source of vitamin C, folate, and potassium. They have a sweet, juicy flavor and pair well with other fruits like strawberries and mango.

Lemons: Lemons are a good source of vitamin C and are known for their cleansing and detoxifying properties. They have a tangy, sour flavor and can be added to smoothies with other fruits or mixed with honey and ginger for a refreshing drink.

Limes: Limes are similar to lemons in taste and nutritional value. They are a good source of vitamin C and can add a zesty flavor to smoothies.

Grapefruits: Grapefruits are rich in vitamin C and fiber, and have been shown to have anti-cancer properties. They have a tart, slightly bitter flavor that pairs well with sweet fruits like pineapple and mango.

Tangerines: Tangerines are a good source of vitamin C and are known for their sweet, juicy flavor. They can be peeled and added to smoothies whole or blended with other fruits like bananas and mango.

When using citrus fruits in smoothies, it's important to remove the seeds and any white pith, which can add a bitter taste. You can also pair citrus fruits with sweeter fruits or honey to balance out their tart flavor.

Chapter four

Turmeric

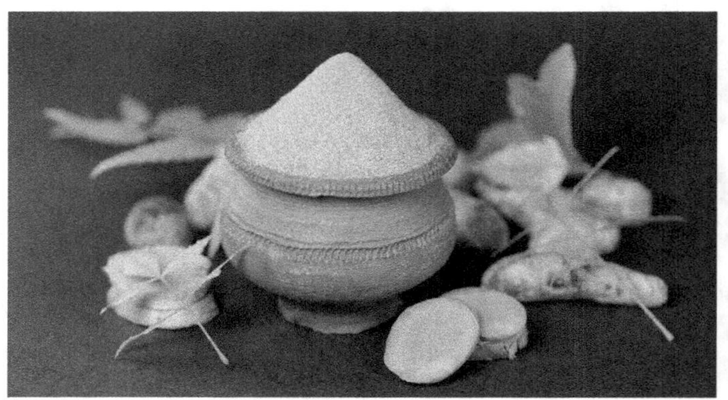

How turmeric contains a compound

called curcumin that has

anti-inflammatory and anti-cancer

properties

Turmeric has been used in traditional medicine for countless years due to its anti-inflammatory and antioxidant properties. A substance known as curcumin, which is the primary active component in turmeric, is in charge of many of its health advantages, including its anti-inflammatory and anti-cancer characteristics.

Curcumin acts by lessening bodily inflammation. The immune system's normal reaction to damage or infection is inflammation, but persistent inflammation may result in a number of disorders, including cancer. It has been shown that curcumin inhibits the action of molecules like cytokines and nuclear factor-kappa B (NF-kB), which are responsible for inflammation in the body.

Additionally discovered to have anti-cancer properties is curcumin. By focusing on several pathways involved in the growth and spread of cancer, it may prevent the growth and spread of cancer cells. Curcumin has been proven to block the action of enzymes that support the growth of cancer cells, cause apoptosis (programmed cell death) in cancer cells, and limit the development of blood vessels that nourish tumors.

Curcumin has been discovered to provide other health advantages in addition to its anti-inflammatory and anti-cancer characteristics. It may enhance cognitive performance, decrease the risk of heart disease, and lessen the signs and symptoms of anxiety and depression.

Despite having only 2-5% curcumin, turmeric can still be a valuable addition to your diet due to its numerous health advantages. It's vital to note that curcumin cannot be absorbed by the body on its own; thus, it is advised to combine turmeric with black pepper, which includes a substance called piperine that may increase curcumin absorption by up to 2000%.

Ways to incorporate turmeric into smoothies

Turmeric can be a great addition to your smoothies, adding a spicy and earthy flavor, as well as its many health benefits. Here are some ways to incorporate turmeric into your smoothies:

Fresh turmeric root: Fresh turmeric root can be found in many grocery stores and health food stores. You can grate or chop a small piece of turmeric root and add it to your smoothie for a fresh and earthy flavor.

Ground turmeric powder: Ground turmeric powder is a more convenient option and can be found in most grocery stores. You can add a teaspoon or two of ground turmeric to your smoothie for a more concentrated dose of curcumin.

Turmeric paste: Turmeric paste is a mixture of ground turmeric, black pepper, and water that has been cooked into a paste. You can make your own turmeric paste or purchase it pre-made. Add a spoonful of turmeric paste to your smoothie for a spicy and aromatic flavor.

Golden milk: Golden milk is a traditional Indian drink made with turmeric, milk, and spices like cinnamon and ginger. You can blend golden milk with frozen bananas and other fruits to make a delicious and healthy smoothie.

Turmeric smoothie cubes: You can make turmeric smoothie cubes by blending fresh turmeric root, black pepper, and coconut milk, and freezing the mixture in ice cube trays. Add a few turmeric smoothie cubes to your smoothie for a spicy and refreshing flavor.

When using turmeric in your smoothies, it's important to pair it with other flavorful ingredients to balance out its earthy taste. Some good pairing options include ginger, cinnamon, honey, coconut milk, and citrus fruits like lemon and orange. Don't forget to add black pepper to help increase the absorption of curcumin in the body.

Ginger

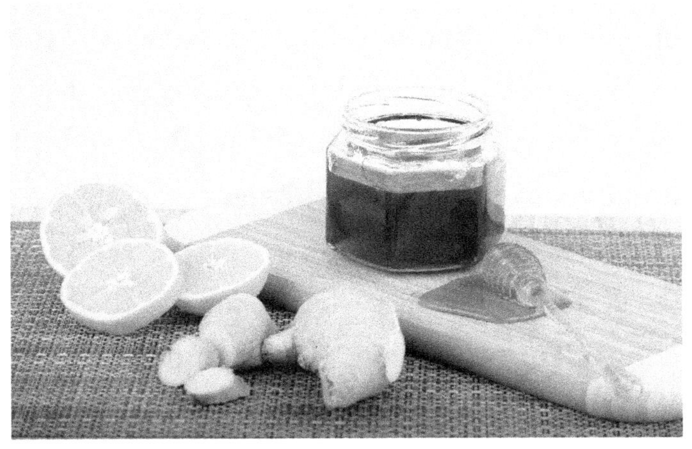

how ginger contains compounds that have been shown to have anti-cancer effects

Ginger is a root that has been used in traditional medicine for thousands of years for its many health benefits. Ginger contains several bioactive compounds, including gingerols, shogaols, and paradols, which have been shown to have anti-cancer effects.

One way that ginger can help prevent cancer is by reducing inflammation in the body. The onset and spread of cancer may be aided by chronic inflammation. Gingerols, which are the main active compounds in ginger, has been shown to inhibit the production of inflammatory molecules in the body, such as cytokines and chemokines.

Gingerols have also been found to have antioxidant properties, which can help protect cells from damage caused by free radicals. Free radicals are unstable molecules that can damage cells and DNA, potentially leading to cancer.

In addition to its anti-inflammatory and antioxidant properties, ginger has been found to have other cancer-fighting properties. It can inhibit the growth and spread of cancer cells by targeting multiple pathways involved in the development and progression of cancer. Gingerols have been shown to induce apoptosis (programmed cell death) in cancer cells, prevent the formation of blood vessels that supply tumors, and inhibit the activity of enzymes that promote the growth of cancer cells.

Furthermore, ginger has been found to enhance the efficacy of chemotherapy and radiation therapy. In one study, patients with advanced colorectal cancer who received ginger supplements along with chemotherapy had a significantly higher survival rate than those who received chemotherapy alone.

Overall, the anti-cancer properties of ginger are due to its ability to reduce inflammation, protect cells from damage, and inhibit the growth and spread of cancer cells. Incorporating ginger into your diet, such as in smoothies, can be a delicious way to take advantage of these health benefits.

Ways to incorporate ginger into smoothies

Ginger is a versatile ingredient that can add a spicy and refreshing flavor to your smoothies, as well as its many health benefits. Here are some ways to incorporate ginger into your smoothies:

Fresh ginger root: Fresh ginger root can be found in most grocery stores and health food stores. You can grate or chop a small piece of ginger root and add it to your smoothie for a fresh and zesty flavor.

Ground ginger powder: Ground ginger powder is a more convenient option and can be found in most grocery stores. You can add a teaspoon or two of ground ginger to your smoothie for a more concentrated dose of gingerol.

Ginger juice: Ginger juice is a more potent option and can be found in some health food stores. You can add a tablespoon or two of ginger juice to your smoothie for a quick and easy boost of flavor and health benefits.

Ginger tea: Ginger tea is a traditional remedy for digestive issues and can also add a spicy and aromatic flavor to your smoothie. Brew a cup of ginger tea, let it cool, and add it to your smoothie along with other ingredients.

Ginger smoothie cubes: You can make ginger smoothie cubes by blending fresh ginger root with water, pouring the mixture into ice cube trays, and freezing it. Add a few ginger smoothie cubes to your smoothie for a refreshing and zesty flavor.

When using ginger in your smoothies, it's important to balance out its strong and spicy flavor with other ingredients. Some good pairing options include citrus fruits, such as lemon and orange, coconut milk, honey, and cinnamon. Ginger also pairs well with other anti-inflammatory and antioxidant ingredients, such as turmeric and blueberries.

Gree Tea

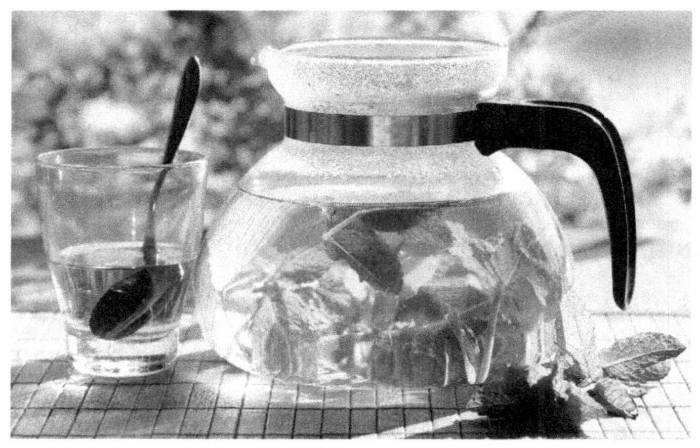

How green tea contains compounds that have been shown to have anti-cancer effects

Green tea is made from the leaves of the Camellia sinensis plant and has been used for centuries in traditional medicine for its many health benefits. Green tea contains several bioactive compounds, including polyphenols, catechins, and flavonoids, which have been shown to have anti-cancer effects.

One of the main polyphenols in green tea is epigallocatechin gallate (EGCG), which has been extensively studied for its anti-cancer properties. EGCG has been found to inhibit the growth and spread of cancer cells in several types of cancer, including breast, prostate, lung, and colon cancer.

EGCG and other green tea polyphenols have been found to work in several ways to help prevent cancer. They can act as antioxidants, protecting cells from damage caused by free radicals, which can contribute to the development of cancer. Green tea polyphenols have also been found to have anti-inflammatory effects, which can help reduce the risk of cancer development.

Green tea polyphenols have also been shown to suppress the action of enzymes that aid in the growth of cancer cells, cause apoptosis (programmed cell death) in cancer cells, and limit the development of blood vessels that nourish tumors.

Studies have also shown that green tea can enhance the efficacy of chemotherapy and radiation therapy in cancer treatment. Green tea polyphenols have been found to sensitize cancer cells to chemotherapy and radiation therapy, making them more effective in killing cancer cells.

Overall, the anti-cancer properties of green tea are due to its high content of polyphenols, particularly EGCG, which can act as antioxidants, anti-inflammatory agents, and anti-cancer agents. Drinking green tea regularly, or incorporating it into your diet through smoothies or other recipes, can be a delicious way to take advantage of these health benefits.

Ways to incorporate green tea into smoothies

Green tea can be a great addition to your smoothies, as it adds a boost of antioxidants and may help reduce the risk of cancer. Here are some ways to incorporate green tea into your smoothies:

Brewed green tea: One simple way to add green tea to your smoothie is to brew a cup of green tea and let it cool. You can then use the tea as the liquid base for your smoothie, instead of using water or milk.

Matcha powder: Matcha is a type of green tea that has been ground into a fine powder. You can add a teaspoon or two of matcha powder to your smoothie for a concentrated dose of antioxidants and a vibrant green color.

Frozen green tea cubes: Brew a cup of green tea and let it cool, then pour it into an ice cube tray and freeze. You can add a few green tea cubes to your smoothie for a refreshing and antioxidant-packed boost.

Green tea extract: Green tea extract is a concentrated form of the beneficial compounds found in green tea. You can add a small amount of green tea extract to your smoothie for a more potent dose of antioxidants.

Pre-made green tea smoothie mix: Some health food stores sell pre-made green tea smoothie mixes that you can simply blend with your other smoothie ingredients for a quick and easy boost of antioxidants.

When using green tea in your smoothies, it's important to balance out its slightly bitter taste with other ingredients. Some good pairing options include citrus fruits, honey, pineapple, and berries. Green tea also pairs well with other antioxidant-rich ingredients, such as spinach and kale.

Garlic

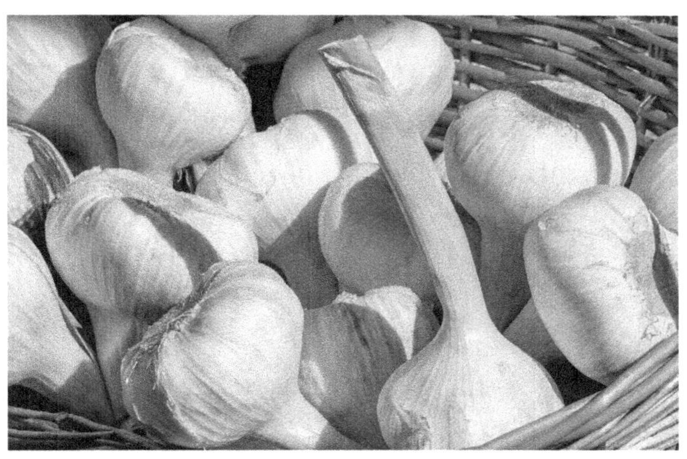

How garlic contains compounds that have been shown to have anti-cancer effects

Garlic is a flavorful ingredient that has been used for centuries in traditional medicine for its many health benefits. Garlic contains several compounds that are believed to have anti-cancer effects, including allyl sulfur compounds and flavonoids. These compounds have been shown to help prevent the formation and growth of cancer cells by inducing cell death, inhibiting cell proliferation, and blocking the formation of blood vessels that tumors need to grow.

One of the key compounds in garlic is allicin, which is responsible for its distinctive smell and flavor. Allicin is released when garlic is chopped or crushed and has been shown to have potent anti-cancer effects in animal and laboratory studies. Allicin and other sulfur compounds in garlic may also help reduce inflammation, another factor that is believed to contribute to the development of cancer.

Research suggests that regular consumption of garlic may help reduce the risk of several types of cancer, including stomach, colon, esophageal, and breast cancer. However, more research is needed to fully understand the mechanisms by which garlic and its compounds exert their anti-cancer effects.

Overall, incorporating garlic into your diet may be a simple and flavorful way to potentially reduce your risk of cancer and promote overall health.

Ways to incorporate garlic into smoothies

Garlic can add a pungent and savory flavor to your smoothies, along with its potential anti-cancer properties. Here are a few ways to incorporate garlic into your smoothies:

Raw garlic: The easiest way to add garlic to your smoothie is to use a fresh garlic clove. Simply peel and chop the garlic, then add it to your blender along with your other ingredients. Start with a small amount, such as half a clove, and adjust to taste.

Roasted garlic: Roasting garlic mellows its flavor and makes it sweeter. To roast garlic, cut off the top of a whole garlic bulb, drizzle with olive oil, and roast in the oven until soft and caramelized. You can then add the roasted garlic cloves to your smoothie for a subtle and sweet garlic flavor.

If you don't have any fresh garlic on hand, you may use garlic powder. For a fast and simple method to add a garlic taste to your smoothie, sprinkle a little garlic powder on top.

Garlic-infused oil: Garlic-infused oil can add a subtle garlic flavor to your smoothie without the pungency of raw garlic. Simply heat the olive oil with a few cloves of crushed garlic until fragrant, then strain out the garlic and use the infused oil in your smoothie.

When using garlic in your smoothies, keep in mind that its flavor can be strong and overpowering. Start with a tiny quantity and titrate to taste is the best approach.

Garlic pairs well with savory ingredients such as spinach, avocado, and cucumber, and can also be balanced with sweet fruits such as berries and bananas.

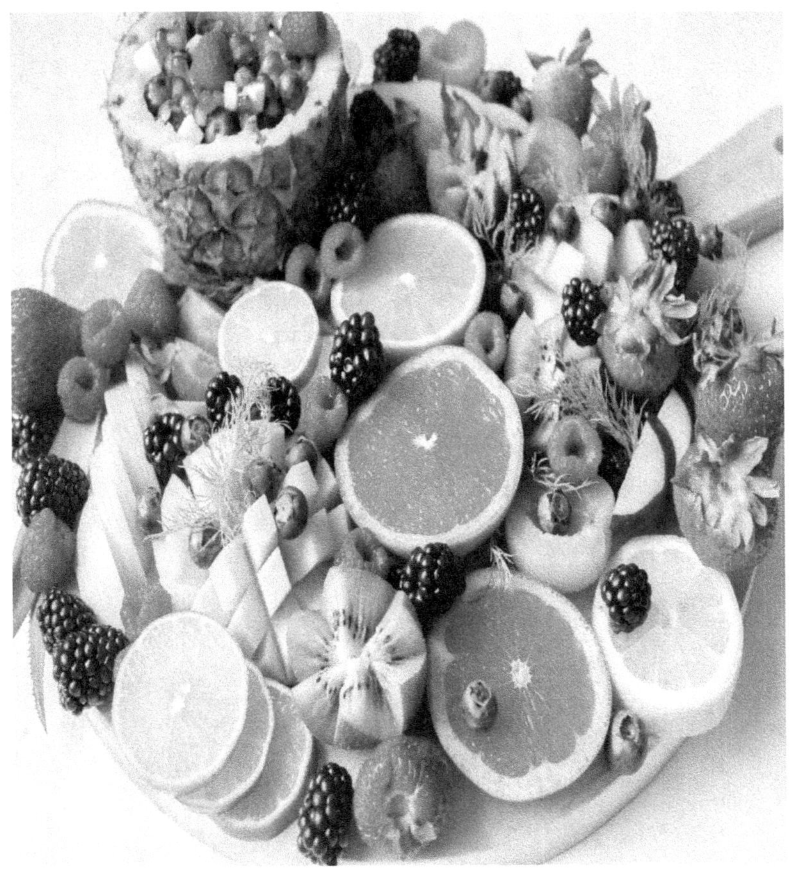

CHAPTER FIVE

Avocado

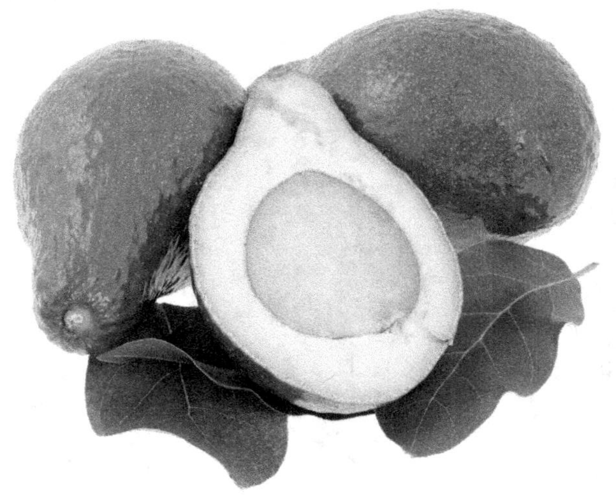

How avocados contain compounds that have been shown to have anti-cancer effects

Avocado is a fruit that is packed with nutrients and has been associated with many health benefits, including potential anti-cancer effects. Avocados contain several bioactive compounds, such as carotenoids, tocopherols, and polyphenols, which have been shown to have anti-cancer properties.

One of the key compounds in avocados is called persenone A, which has been shown to inhibit the growth of cancer cells in laboratory studies. Additionally, avocados are a rich source of monounsaturated fats and dietary fiber, which have been linked to a lower risk of several types of cancer, including colon, breast, and pancreatic cancer.

Studies have also suggested that avocados may have anti-inflammatory effects, which could contribute to their potential anti-cancer properties. Chronic inflammation is a known risk factor for cancer development, and reducing inflammation may help prevent the formation and growth of cancer cells.

While more research is needed to fully understand the mechanisms by which avocados and their compounds exert their anti-cancer effects, incorporating this fruit into your diet may be a simple and delicious way to promote overall health and potentially reduce your risk of cancer.

Ways to incorporate avocado into smoothies

Avocado is a creamy and nutritious ingredient that can add richness and healthy fats to your smoothies. Here are a few ways to incorporate avocado into your smoothies:

Avocado smoothie base: One of the simplest ways to use avocado in a smoothie is to use it as a base. Simply blend a ripe avocado with some almond milk, yogurt, or other liquid of your choice to create a creamy base for your smoothie.

Chocolate avocado smoothie: Avocado pairs well with chocolate, and adding some cocoa powder or chocolate protein powder to your avocado smoothie can create a rich and indulgent treat.

Green smoothie: Avocado can add a creamy texture to green smoothies, which typically include leafy greens like spinach or kale, along with fruits like bananas and berries. Try blending a ripe avocado with some spinach, pineapple, and coconut water for a refreshing and healthy green smoothie.

Berry avocado smoothie: Avocado can also add a creamy texture to berry smoothies, which typically include frozen berries like strawberries, raspberries, or blueberries. Try blending a ripe avocado with some mixed berries, almond milk, and a touch of honey for a sweet and satisfying smoothie.

When using avocado in your smoothies, keep in mind that a little goes a long way. Using too much avocado can make your smoothie too thick and heavy. Start with a quarter to half an avocado and adjust to taste.

Nuts and Seeds

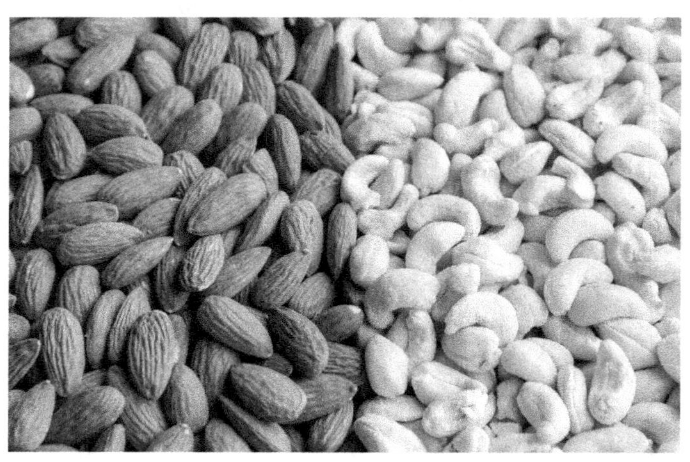

How nuts and seeds contain compounds that helps to prevent cancer

Nuts and seeds are rich in several bioactive compounds, including vitamins, minerals, dietary fiber, and healthy fats, which have been associated with numerous health benefits, including potential anti-cancer effects.

One of the key compounds found in nuts and seeds is phytosterols, which are plant-based compounds that have been shown to have anti-cancer properties. Phytosterols have a similar structure to cholesterol and can help reduce the absorption of cholesterol in the gut, which can help reduce the risk of certain types of cancer, such as colon cancer.

Nuts and seeds also contain antioxidants such as vitamin E, selenium, and flavonoids, which can help protect cells from oxidative stress and DNA damage, both of which are risk factors for cancer. Additionally, nuts and seeds are rich in dietary fiber, which can help reduce inflammation and improve gut health, both of which are important factors in reducing the risk of cancer.

Some specific nuts and seeds have been studied for their potential anti-cancer effects. For example, flaxseeds contain lignans, which have been shown to reduce the risk of breast cancer. Similarly, walnuts contain omega-3 fatty acids, which have been linked to a lower risk of breast and colon cancer.

Overall, incorporating a variety of nuts and seeds into your diet can provide a range of beneficial compounds that may help reduce the risk of cancer and promote overall health.

Specific nuts and seeds to include in smoothies

Nuts and seeds are a great addition to smoothies, as they can provide a range of health benefits, including potential anti-cancer effects. Here are some specific nuts and seeds that you can include in your smoothies:

Chia seeds: Chia seeds are rich in fiber, omega-3 fatty acids, and antioxidants. They can help reduce inflammation and promote gut health. Try adding a tablespoon or two of chia seeds to your smoothie.

Flaxseeds: Flaxseeds are also rich in fiber, omega-3 fatty acids, and lignans, which have been shown to have anti-cancer effects, especially in breast cancer. Try adding a tablespoon of ground flaxseeds to your smoothie.

Almonds: Almonds are a good source of vitamin E, fiber, and healthy fats, which have been associated with reduced risk of cancer. Try adding a handful of almonds or a tablespoon of almond butter to your smoothie.

Hemp seeds: Hemp seeds are a good source of protein, fiber, and omega-3 fatty acids. They can help reduce inflammation and improve heart health. Try adding a tablespoon or two of hemp seeds to your smoothie.

Walnuts: Walnuts are rich in omega-3 fatty acids, antioxidants, and fiber, which have been associated with reduced risk of cancer. Try adding a handful of walnuts or a tablespoon of walnut butter to your smoothie.

When incorporating nuts and seeds into your smoothies, it's important to remember that they are calorie-dense, so it's best to use them in moderation. Try adding a variety of nuts and seeds to your smoothies to maximize their health benefits.

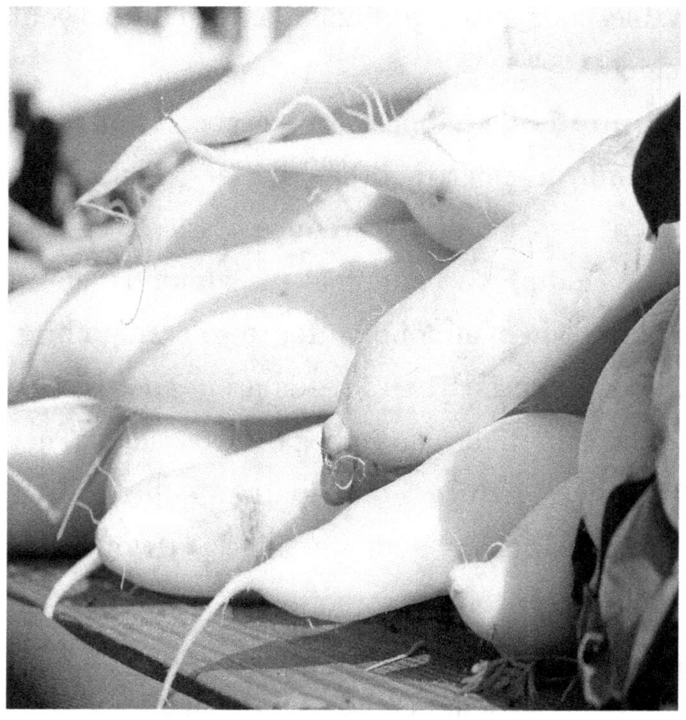

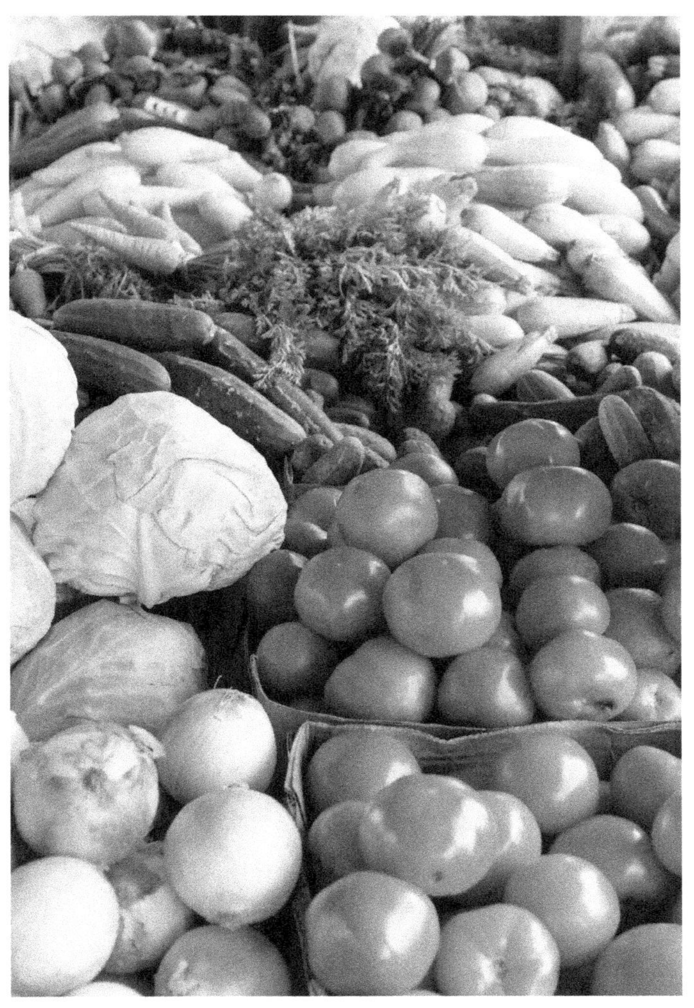

CHAPTER SIX

Dark Chocolate

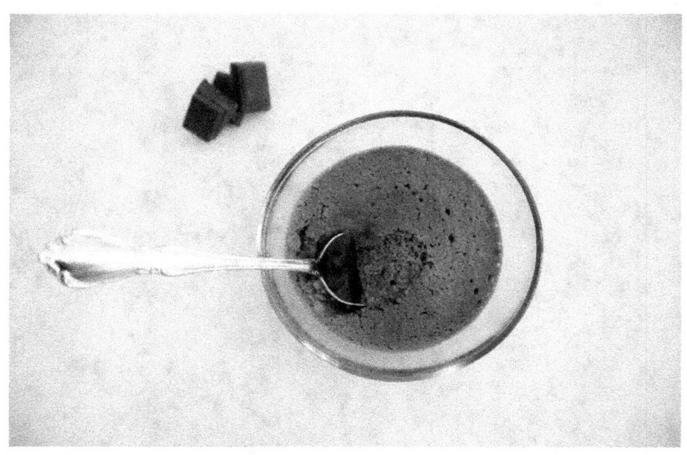

How dark chocolate contains compounds that helps to prevent cancer

Dark chocolate contains several compounds that have been shown to have potential anti-cancer effects. One of the key compounds found in dark chocolate is flavonoids, which are a type of antioxidant that can help protect cells from oxidative stress and DNA damage, both of which are risk factors for cancer.

Flavonoids have been shown to inhibit the growth of cancer cells and induce cancer cell death in laboratory studies. In addition, some studies have suggested that flavonoids may help prevent the formation of new blood vessels that supply tumors with nutrients, thereby slowing or preventing tumor growth.

Dark chocolate also contains other potentially beneficial compounds, such as theobromine, which has been shown to inhibit the growth of breast cancer cells, and resveratrol, which has been shown to have anti-cancer effects in laboratory studies.

It's important to note that not all chocolate is created equal when it comes to potential health benefits. Dark chocolate, which contains a higher percentage of cocoa solids, is generally considered to be healthier than milk chocolate or white chocolate, which contains less cocoa solids and more sugar and milk.

Overall, while more research is needed to fully understand the potential anti-cancer effects of dark chocolate, it's clear that dark chocolate contains several compounds that have been associated with cancer prevention and may be a healthy addition to your diet in moderation.

Ways to incorporate dark chocolate into Smoothies

Incorporating dark chocolate into your smoothies can be a tasty way to add some potential anti-cancer benefits to your diet. Here are a few ways to add dark chocolate to your smoothies:

Use cocoa powder: Cocoa powder is a convenient way to add the chocolate flavor and antioxidants found in dark chocolate to your smoothies. Try adding a tablespoon or two of unsweetened cocoa powder to your smoothie.

Add chocolate chips: For a more indulgent treat, add a handful of dark chocolate chips to your smoothie. Be sure to choose dark chocolate chips with a high percentage of cocoa solids for maximum health benefits.

Make a chocolate sauce: Blend melted dark chocolate with a little milk or cream to make a chocolate sauce that you can swirl into your smoothie. This is a great way to add a rich chocolate flavor to your smoothie.

Use a chocolate protein powder: There are many protein powders on the market that are flavored with chocolate and contain added cocoa powder. Look for a high-quality protein powder with minimal added sugars for maximum health benefits.

When adding dark chocolate to your smoothies, keep in mind that it can be high in calories and fat. Use it in moderation and choose high-quality, dark chocolate with a high percentage of cocoa solids for maximum health benefits.

Beets

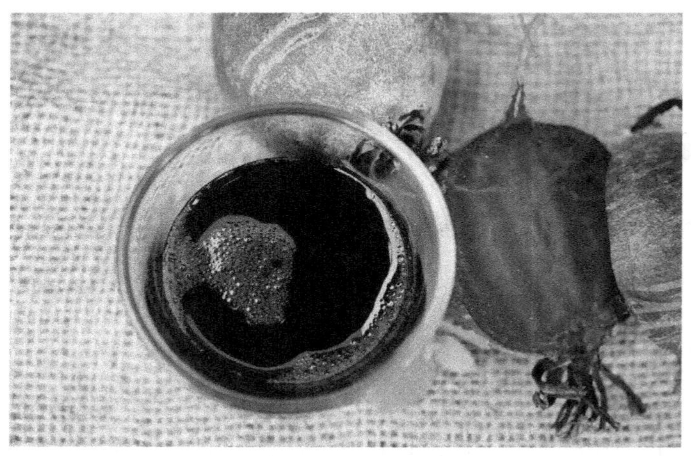

How beets contain compounds that helps to prevent cancer

Beets are a rich source of several compounds that have been shown to have potential anti-cancer effects. One of the most important compounds found in beets is betalain, which is responsible for the vegetable's vibrant red color. Betalains are powerful antioxidants that can help protect cells from oxidative stress and DNA damage, which are risk factors for cancer.

Studies have suggested that betalains may have anti-cancer properties by inhibiting the growth of cancer cells and inducing cancer cell death. In addition, beets are a rich source of dietary nitrates, which can help improve blood flow and reduce inflammation. Chronic inflammation is a risk factor for cancer, and reducing inflammation in the body may help lower the risk of cancer.

Additionally, beets are a good source of fiber, which is necessary for a healthy digestive system. A healthy digestive system is essential for overall health and may play a role in cancer prevention.

Overall, while more research is needed to fully understand the potential anti-cancer effects of beets, they are nutritious vegetable that may offer several health benefits, including potential cancer prevention.

Ways to incorporate beets into smoothies

Beets are a nutritious vegetable that can be a great addition to your smoothies. Here are a few ways to incorporate beets into your smoothie recipes:

Use cooked beets: You can use cooked beets in your smoothies for a sweeter taste and smoother texture. Simply roast or boil beets until they are soft, and then peel and chop them into small pieces before adding them to your smoothie.

Use raw beets: Raw beets are also great in smoothies, but they can be a bit tougher to blend. Try grating the beets or cutting them into small pieces before blending them to help them blend more easily.

Combine with fruits: Beets pair well with sweet fruits like berries, pineapple, and mango. Try adding a handful of these fruits to your smoothie along with the beets for a delicious and nutritious combination.

Add some greens: If you want to boost the nutritional value of your smoothie, add some leafy greens like spinach, kale, or chard to the mix. Greens are packed with vitamins and minerals and can help balance out the sweetness of the beets.

Experiment with flavors: Beets have a distinct earthy flavor that may not be everyone's cup of tea. Try adding other ingredients like ginger, lemon, or mint to your smoothie to create a flavor profile that you enjoy.

Overall, beets are a versatile and nutritious vegetable that can add a pop of color and flavor to your smoothies. Experiment with different ingredients and flavor combinations to find a recipe that works for you.

Tomatoes

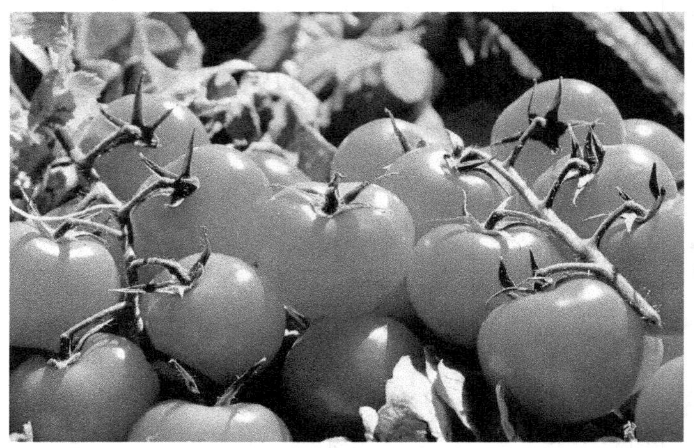

How tomatoes contain compounds that helps to prevent cancer

Ways to incorporate tomatoes into smoothies

Tomatoes are a rich source of several compounds that have been shown to have potential anti-cancer effects. One of the most important compounds found in tomatoes is lycopene, which is a powerful antioxidant that can help protect cells from oxidative damage. Oxidative damage is a risk factor for cancer, and reducing this damage may help lower the risk of cancer.

Studies have suggested that lycopene may have anti-cancer properties by inhibiting the growth of cancer cells and inducing cancer cell death. In addition, tomatoes are a good source of other antioxidants, including vitamins A and C, which can also help protect cells from damage.

Tomatoes are also rich in fiber, which is important for maintaining a healthy digestive system. A healthy digestive system is essential for overall health and may play a role in cancer prevention.

Overall, while more research is needed to fully understand the potential anti-cancer effects of tomatoes, they are a nutritious food that may offer several health benefits, including potential cancer prevention.

Ways to incorporate tomatoes into your smoothies

Use fresh or canned tomatoes: You can use fresh or canned tomatoes in your smoothies. If you're using fresh tomatoes, remove the stem and core before adding them to your blender. If you're using canned tomatoes, drain them and rinse them before adding them to your blender.

Combine with other fruits and vegetables: Tomatoes pair well with other fruits and vegetables like cucumbers, peppers, and citrus fruits. Try adding a variety of colorful produce to your smoothie for a nutritious and flavorful drink.

Use tomato juice: If you don't have fresh or canned tomatoes on hand, you can use tomato juice as a base for your smoothie. Look for a low-sodium or no-salt-added tomato juice for the healthiest option.

Add herbs and spices: Tomatoes pair well with herbs and spices like basil, oregano, and black pepper. Try adding a pinch of these seasonings to your tomato smoothie for added flavor and nutrition.

Overall, there are many creative ways to incorporate tomatoes into your smoothies. Experiment with different ingredients and flavor combinations to find a recipe that works for you.

Conclusion

In conclusion, incorporating cancer-fighting ingredients into your diet, including in smoothies, can be a delicious and easy way to promote optimal health and potentially reduce your risk of cancer. The 15 ingredients discussed in this conversation, including berries, leafy greens, cruciferous vegetables, citrus fruits, turmeric, ginger, green tea, garlic, avocado, nuts, seeds, dark chocolate, beets, tomatoes, and carrots, have all been shown to have potential cancer-fighting properties. However, it's important to remember that no single food or ingredient can prevent or cure cancer on its own and that a healthy and balanced diet, regular exercise, and other healthy lifestyle choices are all important for reducing your cancer risk and promoting overall health. So, incorporate these cancer-fighting ingredients into your smoothies and focus on overall healthy lifestyle habits for optimal health.

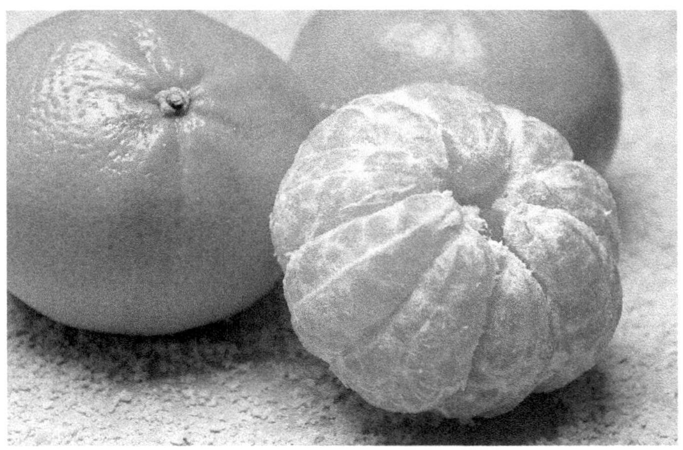

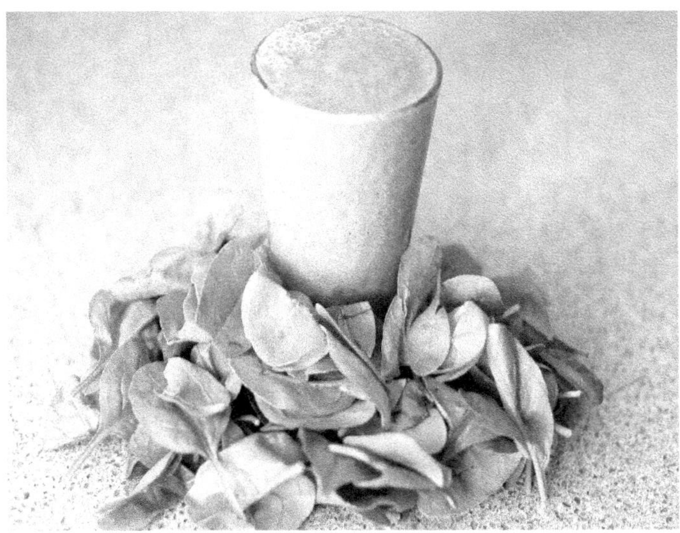